I AM FITNESS!

By Karen Dennis

Publishing services provided by HelaWrite LLC
& EPIC Books Publishing Indie Division

Edited and formatted by Tamar Hela

Summary:
Karen Dennis, a certified fitness professional of twenty-
one years, is the owner of Karen Dennis Power Trainer
Studio. She is a graduate of Integrative Institute of
Nutrition and is a Board certified Holistic Health
Practitioner, certified raw vegan chef, personal trainer,
wife, mother of five, and grandmother of two. Karen
wrote *I AM FITNESS!* in hopes of helping you achieve
your daily goals and ultimate happiness. Inside, you'll
find quick results-oriented workouts, nutritional tips,
and motivational quotes. Keep this book handy in your
pocket or gym bag and get ready to be inspired while
achieving your fitness goals.

[Non-Fiction-General, Non-Fiction-Fitness, Non-
Fiction-Inspirational]

ISBN-10: 1941077048
ISBN-13: 978-1-941077-04-7

"I believe that the very purpose of life is to be happy. From the very core of our being, we desire contentment. In my own limited experience I have found that the more we care for the happiness of others, the greater is our own sense of well-being. Cultivating a close, warmhearted feeling for others automatically puts the mind at ease. It helps remove whatever fears or insecurities we may have and gives us the strength to cope with any obstacles we encounter. It is the principal source of success in life. Since we are not solely material creatures, it is a mistake to place all our hopes for happiness on external development alone. The key is to develop inner peace."

~ Dalai Lama

About

My name is Karen Dennis. I have been a fitness professional for 21 years. I'm a mother of five, and a grandmother of two. At 48 years old, I am a health nutritional coach, a vegan, a certified raw vegan chef, personal trainer, and the owner of Karen Dennis Power Trainer Studio.

I wrote this pocket-sized booklet in hopes of helping you achieve your daily goals and ultimate happiness. It has my greatest, quickest, and most-guaranteed, results-oriented workouts for your legs, arms, back, and abs. These workouts require your body weight and a little bit of equipment. I've added some tips to keep you focused, motivated, and hyped—all while being exposed to some great nutritional tips. We all know that just working out won't work. YOU CANNOT OUT-TRAIN A BAD DIET!

Tip #1

LET YOUR FOOD BE YOUR MEDICINE

Every piece of food that goes in your mouth should be viewed as:

- Is this going to bring health and healing to my body?

- Is this food going to inflame my midsection, make my arms more or less toned, and add to my thighs?

- Or is this food going to energize me?

- Is it going to keep me looking and feeling like I'm on top of the world, while having a better quality of life?

- And will I be able to fit into my jeans?

Tip #2

EAT YOUR HEAVIEST MEALS EARLY

Cut off all heavy eating by 7 p.m. Try eating your largest meals early in the day, while you're up and moving. This way, when your body starts to come down and you're feeling tired, you won't have a full stomach before going to bed.

You should always go to bed *at least* two hours after your last meal. NEVER go to bed on a full stomach.

Tip# 3

SECONDARY FOODS

When you go shopping for produce—secondary foods—shop for the colors of the rainbow. I love to pick different colors of produce when I'm shopping. Each one of the colors represents a different nutritional value:

Red – Helps to protect against cancers of the lung, colon, esophagus, breast, and skin.

Blue - Good for lowering the risk of heart disease, prevents age-related memory loss, and keeps the eyes and urinary tract healthy.

White - May lower the risk of heart disease, and helps to ease the symptoms of allergies like hay fever.

Purple - Good for lowering the risk of gum disease and stomach ulcers.

I AM FITNESS!

Green - Excellent for improving blood circulation, lowering cholesterol, kidney function, vision, and clearing congestion.

Yellow - Promotes collagen formation and healthy joints; encourages alkaline balance.

Orange - Works to build healthy bones, and fights free radicals.

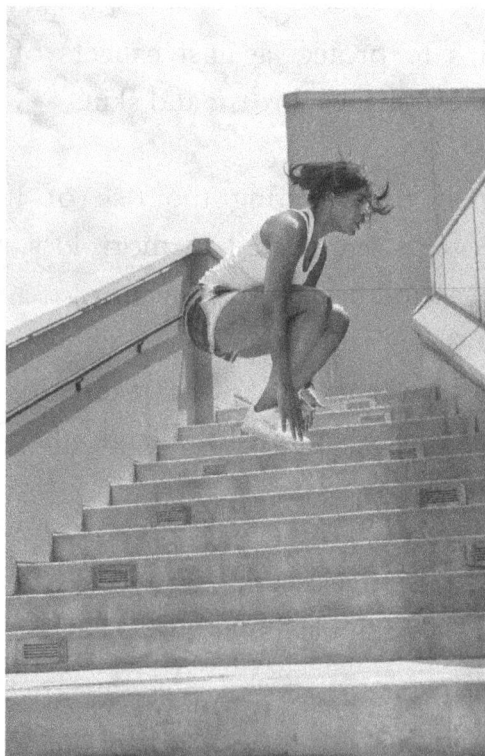

Tip #4

SLIM WAISTLINE WORKOUT PART 1

STATIONARY LUNGES WITH A TWIST AND SMALL A MEDICINE BALL

- Right foot forward, left foot back, raised up on the ball of your foot, both knees are bent at a 90-degree angle
- With both arms extended, holding the ball, twist towards your right side, hold for a slight pause, and start from the beginning
- 128 repetitions, each side

STANDING K

- Just like the letter K, lift your left arm up overhead, right arm holding 2-lb. weight
- Slightly bend the left standing leg, while the right arm and leg move toward each other
- Bend your torso while moving your right leg and arm
- 128 repetitions, each side

Tip #5

A PERFECTED SILHOUETTE WORKOUT

- Use a 5-minute song for slow and controlled lunges, or do 128 repetitions for each leg

- 128 repetitions rectus abs small crunches

- 128 repetitions pelvic thrusts

- 128 repetitions bicycles

- 5-minute planks with alternating leg lifts

BACK EXTENSION

- Lying face down, balls of the feet remain on the floor, thighs off the floor, and hands under the chin

- Lift the upper body for 128 repetitions in slow and controlled movements

I AM FITNESS!

ALTERNATING ARMS AND BACK SWIMMING EXTENSIONS

- Lying face down on your stomach, alternate opposite arm and leg raises in slow and controlled movements, 128 repetitions

- From the waist down, lift both legs up off the floor; while your chin rests on your hands, engage your core, and constantly contract your gluteal muscles, in slow and controlled movements

PLANKS ALTERNATE SIDE TAPS

- In a plank position, alternate tap up: foot goes towards your elbow and shoulder

- 128 repetitions, or 5 minutes, in slow and controlled movements

- Finish off with dead bugs for 5 minutes, or 128 repetitions

Tip #6

STRENGTHEN/STRETCH YOUR CALVES

This is for all the ladies who complain that they can't walk the next day because of their beautiful, 5-inch stilettos, and yet want to continue to wear them. Here is a workout that will strengthen/stretch your calf muscles:

- Walk on your tippy toes for three of your favorite songs, or do 128 repetitions

- While staying in place, place your feet in a parallel position and move up and down on your tippy toes

- Turn out your feet to first ballet position and move up and down on your tippy toes

- Turn your feet inward (toe-to-toe) and move up and down

- Foam roll the calf muscles and stretch while standing or lying on the floor doing static calf muscle stretch

Tip #7

TRYING TO LOSE THOSE LAST 10-20 POUNDS

Go vegan for two or three months, and your body will shed those pounds for sure. Here's what a typical day/meal plan looks like for me:

- Breakfast: Green smoothie

- Breakfast/Lunch: Zucchini salad with garlic, tomatoes, sautéed spinach with onions, and mushrooms

- Snack: Green smoothie

- Lunch/Dinner: Roasted chickpeas on top of an avocado salad with sprouts, purple cabbage, cucumber, romaine, a sprinkle of chia seeds, and a little mango sauce

- Snack: Green smoothie

- Drink plenty of water throughout the day

- No processed foods, no wine, no alcohol, no sweets, no rice, no potatoes, no grains, no animal meat, no fish, no candy, no chips, no soy, no juice, no diary, and no eggs

- When returning to you regular eating routine, please remember to consume meat 1-2 times per week, but only once in a day

- Always choose organic, grass-fed meats or wild- caught salmon

Tip #8

YOUR BODY LOVES WATER

Drink half your body weight in water, within the 24-hour period of the day, but not all in one hour. You must drink water throughout the day.

<u>For example</u>: If you weigh 200 pounds, you should drink 100 ounces of water a day.

Tip #9

DANCER'S ARMS

Are you tried of arms that are not toned? Try incorporating these workouts:

WITH 3-5 LB. WEIGHTS

- Front arm raises, 32 repetitions x 4 sets
- Side arm raises, 32 repetitions x 4 sets
- Shoulder presses, 32 repetitions x 4 sets
- Elbow-to-elbow, 32 repetitions x 4 sets
- Triceps kickbacks, 32 repetitions x 4 sets

Make sure your elbows remain high, slightly lean forward, bend your knees, keep elbows close to your body, and extend your elbows.

USING YOUR OWN BODY WEIGHT

- Triceps dips, 32 repetitions x 4 sets
- Triceps one-arm dips, 32 repetitions x 4 sets

Tip # 10

SCULPTED FEMININE CHEST

This is a beautiful movement that will keep your arms, chest, back, and core tight.

SWAN DIVES

- In a modified plank position, rise up on your toes, drop your head between your arms, and bend your arms while lowering your chest towards the floor

- Then push up, recover, and repeat

- Do this 32 times to slow and beautiful music

Tip #11

SLIM WAISTLINE WORKOUT PART 2

Here's another workout that will surely help you to slim down your waistline:

- Side-lying crunches on the floor

- 128 repetitions each

- Single extended leg

- Hands behind the head

- Abdominal crunches on the Bosu 128 times

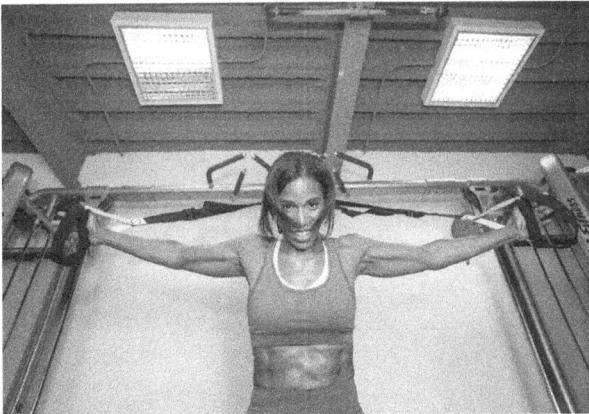

Tip #12

OUTSIDE CARDIO

Every day, walk or jog 20K steps. Get a pedometer and compete with yourself.

- 20K steps are equal to 2K calories that you burn
- 30K steps are equal to 3K calories that you burn
- 35K steps are equal to 3.5K calories that you will burn, which is equal to one pound of fat

Walk 35K steps a day, 5 days a week, and you will drop 5 pounds in a week.

Tip #13

LAUGHTER

I love this tip so much: Laughter! Did you know that laughter helps you to burn calories? I laugh hard and quite often, every day. Sometimes I'll get my favorite DVD and sit and laugh for the length of the DVD.

Laughter, for me, releases all stress. It gives me a playful attitude, more, clarity of thought, and I'm even more loving to my family and friends. Laugh away those pounds.

Tip #14

YOU AND NATURE

Go to the park for a quiet walk. Nature has a beautiful way of reconnecting us to a more relaxed self!

Tip #15

BEING A KID

Do a cartwheel and some handstands. I must tell you that it is so much fun doing a cartwheel. And not only is it fun, but it aggressively engages/works your core/midsection.

Tip #16

SENSUAL LEGS WORKOUT PART 1

If you desire killer legs, then try out this workout that I love:

- You will need three 2-lb. medicine balls

- Lying with your back on the floor, place one ball under each foot, with one ball between the knees

- Place your hands at your side and exhale upon movement

- Lift your gluteus off the floor, hold at the top, release to the ground, and start again

- Repeat 128 times

Tip #17

<u>BOOTY BLAST</u>

- Place the physio ball on the floor, lay on your back, heels on top of the ball, toes pointed up, bend your knees at a 90-degree angle, engage your core

- Lift up your buttocks, and extend your legs out, and return and repeat

- Remain in a bridged position

- Don't let your gluteus touch the floor

Tip #18

<u>BELLY DANCE</u>

Belly Dance for a sensual, challenging workout. Get a Belly Dance scarf—preferably one with coins. Play some beautiful music and dance, incorporating beautiful turns, arm movement, and floor moves.

Tip #19

BALLET WORKS

Try incorporating some ballet moves in your workout. I love working with the bars.

- Place your foot on the highest bar, depending on your height

- With your standing leg and your foot turned out, do a small plissé

- It lengthens and stretches your legs

Tip #20

CELLULITE TERMINATOR WORKOUT PART 1

- 10-20 lb. ankle weights

- Lie on the floor on your side, and lift your leg to the height of your hip

- 32 repetitions, each side

Tip #21

30-MINUTE QUICK BLAST

- 5 minutes with the jump rope (2 lb. weighted rope)
- 2.5 minutes front arm raises (5 lbs.)
- 2.5 minutes side arm raises (5 lbs.)
- 2.5 minutes weighted jump rope
- 5 minutes push-up alternating kicks
- 5 minutes jump tucks
- 5 minutes triceps dips (body weight)
- 2.5 minutes burpees

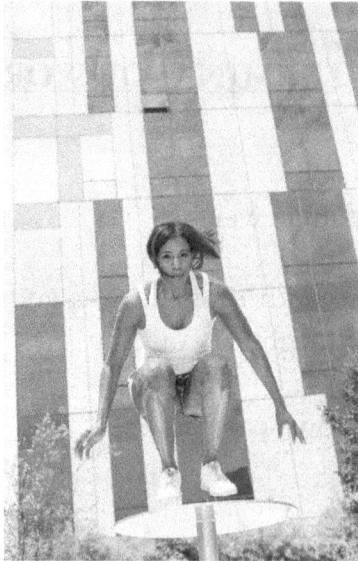

Tip #22

<u>BALANCE, EYES CLOSED</u>

- On the blue side of the Bosu, try to balance yourself with your eyes closed

- When you have mastered the blue side, flip it to the other side for a more challenging core and balance workout

We need balance so we can continually wear our stilettos and not fall.

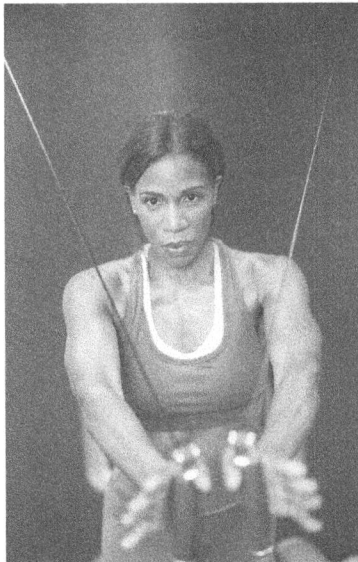

Tip #23

REST DAY

Take one <u>complete</u> rest day!

In the space provided below, take some time to reflect on the healthy habits you've been incorporating for your life. What are changes you've seen? How will you continue to stay positive and motivated?

_____

_____

_____

_____

_____

_____

Tip #24

THE BEST PEDOMETER

Purchase a pedometer for accountability. My favorite is from Amazon.com. The Ormon (blue and silver) costs about $22.00, and I wear mine every day; basic and simple. Be certain that you walk a minimum of 10K steps a day, every day, for the rest of your life.

Tip #25

TRUE BODY FAT

Hydrostatic weighing: If you want to truly know your body fat percentage, then you need to get weighed hydrostatically. There is a company that you can go to, or they can come to you. Visit: www.fitnesswave.com.

Tip #26

TIME IS OF ESSENCE

When you finish working out, it's extremely important to eat. You have 90 minutes until the cells in your body close for your food to aid in muscle rebuilding.

Tip #27

IT'S NEVER TOO LATE—EVERYONE CAN MOVE

Fitness is for everyone. Fitness doesn't discriminate based on age. I treat my senior clients just like I do my non-senior clients. They jump rope, climb the Jacob's ladder, and use the ultra slide. I do modify the workout for them, but it makes them feel young, and accomplished.

Tip #28

MORNING IS THE BEST

It's best to go to the office after you have had a good workout! You have just finished releasing your ENDOMORPHS, which are the natural high releaser, and your thoughts are clearer. If I'm seeking an answer and can't seem to come up with a solution, I pray about it and then I go and work out. It's like the solution is basically already there, and working out aids in bringing it to the forefront. Thank you, GOD, for putting this in us.

Tip #29

GET IT OUT OF THE WAY

Work out in the morning–go hard. Get your fitness routine done early so it's already finished for the day.

Tip #30

NOT CONFINED TO ONE PLACE

Make every opportunity an opportunity to work out. In my home, I always go up the stairs by twos, sometimes I go by threes—it's a great burn. No equipment necessary.

Tip #31

RULES OF ENERGY IN EATING & RULES OF ENERGY OUT MOVEMENT

80/20 percent rule. The rule is that fitness is all about 80% of eating live and clean foods and 20% of movement. You cannot out-train your bad eating habits.

Tip #32

DEEP TISSUE

Find a spa, or massage therapist, and get a monthly deep tissue massage. If you work out everyday, this is mandatory.

Tip #33

FIT CHALLENGES

Enter a fitness challenge—Diva Dash, Iron Man, or Cross Fit—to see how you measure up, and also make new friends.

Tip #34

SUPPORT GROUP

If you are just starting out, surround yourself with a strong support group. Your new family is called your "fitness family."

Tip #35

YOU ARE NOT ALONE

If you are just starting out, you may lose friends. When you begin shedding pounds, chances are that your friends may look at you in another light. It's not that she/he isn't happy for you; it's just that they wish they had the same willpower that you have.

Tip #36

STRIKE A POSE

Document your transformation. Take pictures of yourself every two months in a sports bra, and shorts, with your hair pulled back.

Tip #37

YOUR CLOTHES ARE THE TRUE MEASURE OF WEIGHT LOSS

Don't get caught up with the scale. Fat weighs less than muscle, but takes up more space; whereas muscles weighs more than fat and yet takes up less space. Focus on the inches, and then the weight loss will follow. Muscle burns fat away, to never come back.

Tip #38

IMAGINATION

The art and practice of visualization. Quick story: When I first started out as a fitness instructor, I used to look at the poster that was kept on the aerobics floor. One day, I really studied the picture and thought to myself that I would like to have legs like the ones that were shown in the picture. I had kept that picture in my head, and within six months, I had those legs. So, visualization is extremely powerful.

Tip #39

I LOVE ME SOME ME

How often do you say to yourself that you love yourself? I say it 100 times a day. My body responds so affectionately. It reminds me of hearing my mom say it to me. Always encourage yourself...every day, always.

Tip #40

I'M SO IN LOVE WITH MYSELF

How often do you hug yourself? I hug myself 100 times a day or more. I walk around with the biggest smile ever. Me being in love with myself creates a glow that is illuminated to others.

Tip #41

MIRROR, MIRROR ON THE WALL!

When was the last time you looked in the mirror, with all the lights on, totally naked, and said, "I Love You?" Touch and caress yourself to health, and a better quality of life.

Tip #42

SELFLESSNESS

Pay it forward. This is a huge one. When you reach your goal and you are being loving, and are in love with yourself, it is your destiny to help someone who was once like you. Show them love, compassion, and listen. That's the gift that keeps on giving! A simple act of kindness goes a long way.

Tip #43

CREATE A SLAMMING PLAYLIST!

I mean the one where you are screaming your head off or the kind where you simply must dance, no matter where you are. I LOVE music and have danced from sunrise to sunset. Music is my therapy!

Tip #44

STAYING THE COURSE

Sometimes, the "old person" tries to creep up on us if we are not watching. Don't get in your own way.

Tip #45

IT'S TIME NOW

Elevate yourself by becoming an instructor or personal trainer. If you are interested in becoming an Instructor or Trainer, I would advise that you:

1. Talk to the manager at your local gym

2. Get CPR certified

3. Get Group Instructor certified

4. Get Personal Trainer certified

5. Start

Tip #46

DON'T EVER FORCE YOUR FAMILY MEMBERS TO BE LIKE YOU

Live the lifestyle in front of your family! If your spouse, and children don't work out, don't force them by yelling, taking food away, calling them names, or being disgusted with them. Please remember from where you came from.

I will be the first to say the only way you will win your family over to your side of healthy living is by example. Loving your transformation, and loving them for the beautiful individuals they are. Trust me: they will all come around.

All of my children are extremely fit, and my grandchildren love working out. My granddaughter is a dancer and my grandson loves doing push-ups. Building a legacy of health and wellness is imperative in this day and time.

Tip #47

DON'T FAKE THE FUNK

Remain humble always and do not be intimidating. It's easier to attract flies with honey than with vinegar.

Tip #48

BUILD UP NEVER TEAR DOWN

Never refer to yourself or anyone negatively. Remember: What goes around comes around, and you reap what you sow.

Tip #49

THE ART OF LISTENING

Learn to love to listen to others when they speak.

Tip #50

FUN TIMES

You are in control of your destiny. Fitness is a place where you can find your true self. Have fun learning, changing, and becoming a more loving person.

Tip #51

REMAIN LOVING

Remain true to who you are. As you shed the weight, your alter ego will come out, and it's up to you to make certain that you don't go overboard. A whole different world is going to open up, and my advice is to remain true to who you are!

Tip #52

LIFESTYLE

Try other ways of training: rock climbing, antigravity yoga, pole dancing...just have an open mind to keep it fun, mix it up, and make it challenging.

Tip #53

LOVE YOUR SPINE

- Lie down on the floor on your back, with your legs draped over an ottoman, and close your eyes

- Start by doing 2 minutes

- Progress to 5 minutes

- Then work your way up to 20-30 minutes

Your spine will love you for this. If you have lower back issues, this will help.

Tip #54

TALK TO YOUR DOCTOR

Always consult your doctor on every level of exercise programs you are doing.

Tip #55

COMMUNICATION IS A MUST

If you are on any type of medication and you're thinking about not taking them without your doctor's guidance, please don't do that! Please, please, please, include your doctor. Express to him/her that you would like to wean your way off of them. You will be successful in doing so.

Tip #56

THE ART OF REST

I Love to sleep, I Love to Sleep, I Love to Sleep! Sleep is the only way in which your body breaks down to repair and rebuild yourself.

Listen to me when I say this: No matter how much you work out, you will never be able to burn off fat more than when you are at rest. Your beautiful body burns way more calories at sleep than it does when you're physically active. Growth spurts occur during REM sleep: deep— deep sleep!

Tip #57

HOW MUCH SLEEP DO YOU GET DAILY?

You should sleep at least 7-8 hours in a day. Sleep helps you to lose weight, de-stress, rev up your metabolism, and remain creative.

Tip #58

MOTIVATION

"If we did all the things that we are capable of doing, we would literally astound ourselves."
~ Thomas Edison

Tip #59

ACT NOW

"We live in deeds, not years: In thoughts not breaths; in feelings, not in figures on a dial. We should count time by heart throbs. He most lives who thinks most, feels the noblest, acts the best."
~ David Bailey

Tip #60

YOU ARE YOUR DESTINY

Don't wait for your ship to come in, swim out to it. ~ Anon

Tip #61

TAKE CONTROL

"In essence, if we want to direct our lives, we must take control of our consistent actions. It's not what we do once in a while that shapes our lives, but what we do consistently."
~ Anthony Robbins

Tip #62

SENSUAL LEGS WORKOUT PART 2

- Standing Side Leg Lifts
- Place your hands on your waist, and lift the outside leg, slow and controlled, while engaging your core
- Do 128 repetitions, each leg

Tip #63

SCISSORS

- Lie on the floor, on your back, with 5-lb. ankle weights
- Alternate leg crossover
- 128 repetitions

Tip #64

BUTT TONER

- Rocking Horse: Lie on stomach, legs bent up towards the ceiling at a 90-degree angle; reach arms back to grab each ankle, lift chest and legs and hold for 60 seconds
- Recover and repeat 4 more times

Tip #65

BUTT LIFTER

- Standing side stationary lunges
- 128 repetitions

Tip #66

CELLULITE TERMINATOR WORKOUT PART 2

- Kneeling Side Leg Lifts
- Use a physio ball
- 128 repetitions

Tip #67

<u>STRETCH YOUR CALF MUSCLES</u>

- Place your foam roll under mid calf

- Cross left leg over right leg to increase pressure

- Slowly roll calf area to find most tender spot

- Once it's identified, hold until tenderness reduces (30 seconds minimum)

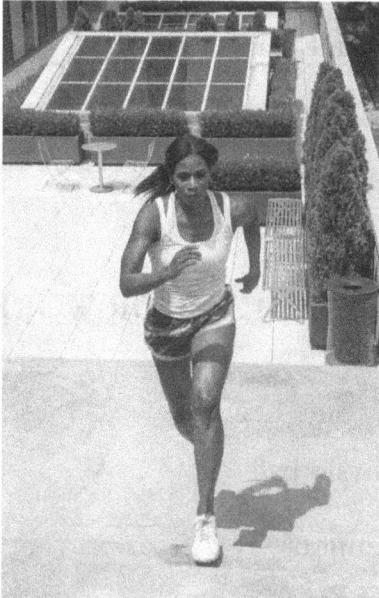

Tip #68

STRETCH YOUR HAMSTRINGS

- Sit with the foam roller under your right thigh

- Place your hands palms own on the floor (fingers towards your body)

- Keep your left foot off the ground by stacking your feet on top of each other (heel of left foot on the toe of the right foot)

- Supporting your body weight with your hands, lift up and roll up and down from your gluteus to the back of your knee

- Repeat on the other side

Tip #69

<u>STRETCH YOUR QUADRICEPS</u>

- Lie face down with the foam roller under your right thigh

- Put your forearm on the ground

- Keep your left foot off the ground by stacking your feet on top of each other (toe of left foot on heel of right foot)

- Supporting your body weight with your forearms, roll up and down from the bottom of the hip to the top of your knees

- Hold for 30 seconds

- Repeat on the other side

Tip #70

STRETCH YOUR INNER THIGHS

- Lie face down with inner thigh flexed and the foam roll towards the groin area, inside the upper thigh

- Slowly roll the inner thigh area to find the most tender spot

- Once located, hold for at least 30 seconds

Tip #71

STRETCH YOUR OUTER THIGHS

- Lie on one side of the foam roll, just in front of the hip

- Cross the top leg over the lower leg, with your foot touching the floor

- Slowly roll from hip joint to outside part of the knee to find the most tender spot

- Once identified, hold the tender spot until the discomfort is released, about 30 seconds

Tip #72

STRETCH YOUR UPPER/LOWER BACK

- Sit on the foam roll and roll down onto your back, while keeping your core engaged
- Slowly move forward and backwards, stretching both your upper and lower back

Tip #73

STRETCH THE MUSCLES AROUND YOUR NECK

- Stand hip-width apart
- Engage your core
- Exhale, relax your shoulders, and slowly pull your head (ear) toward the side of the right shoulder, and repeat on the opposite side
- Hold the stretch for 30 seconds

Tip #74

STRETCH YOUR CHEST MUSCLES

- Stand against an object and form a 90-degree angle with your arm

- Draw in your navel

- Slowly lean forward until a slight stretch is felt in the front shoulder and chest area

- Hold the stretch for 30 seconds

- Repeat on the opposite side

Tip #75

STRETCH YOUR LATISSIMUS DORSI

- Kneel behind the stability ball

- Place your fist, thumb pointed straight up towards the ceiling, inside palm facing you on the ball

- Facing downwards, bend from your waist, flatten your back, and engage your core

- Slowly reach the arm straight out by rolling the ball forward

- Hold the stretch for 30 seconds

DEDICATION

This booklet is dedicated to the loves of my life: Michael Dennis Sr., my husband of 25 years. Our 5 children: Tanihya, Zevenia, Mike Jr., Jamee, and Makenna. Our two grandchildren: Cirriah, and Christopher. My mother: Joan Burton, who introduced me to the WORLD OF DANCE. And to my countless team members currently and long ago: Thank you for entrusting me with your lives.

Thank you, Lila Dennis, for exposing me to this wonderful life of Fitness, Freedom, and Fun, 21 years ago.

I AM FITNESS!

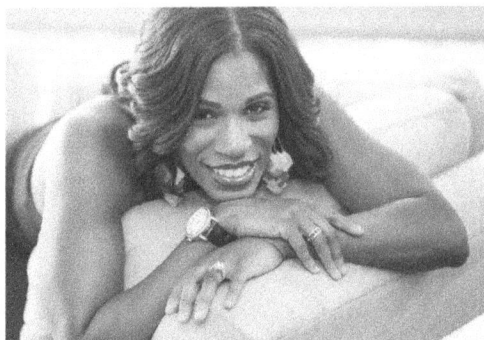

ABOUT THE AUTHOR

Karen Dennis is a Certified Personal Trainer, Master Trainer, and a renowned Power Trainer. I AM FITNESS! is her debut book as a fitness and nutrition author. She finds her inspiration from the Virtuous Woman in Proverbs 31:10, which describes the woman that has it all. Karen doesn't just believe in this for herself; she believes that her clients—and now her readers—can have it all, too.

She has changed the dynamics of the fitness industry. Karen's out-of-the-box training propels her to be one of the best in the business. She expects nothing less than perfection from all her clients, and guarantees long-lasting results.

Through Karen's Power Training, she focuses on four areas: being Spiritually Connected, Emotionally Aligned, Mentally Tough, and Physically Fit. She challenges her clients and readers to move outside their comfort zones, so that they can be someone who has it all.

Find out more about Karen at:

www.karendennis.com

www.ingramcontent.com/pod-product-compliance
Lightning Source LLC
Chambersburg PA
CBHW060636280326
41933CB00012B/2055